MW01291636

Intermittent Fasting Complete Guide for Beginners

How to Lose Weight, Increase Your Energy, Live a Longer and Healthier Life Using the Scientific Phenomenon of Autophagy

May Green

Contents

Text Copyright © May Green

Legal & Disclaimer

Introduction

Thank you for purchasing this book. You have just begun a tremendous journey of revolutionizing your body for better health, better looks, and improved longevity. But since you have just purchased this book, you undoubtedly have some questions about intermittent fasting and whether or not it is really for you.

The truth is that intermittent fasting is not some new starvation fad diet. It is a way of eating that times your food intake to maximize health and weight loss. By playing into your body's natural cycles, intermittent fasting enables you to avoid overeating, burn fat more efficiently, and achieve greater metabolic balance. It is also not the brainchild of some diet fanatic or weight loss guru with no medical degree – it is a tried and true, scientifically-proven way to better manage your diet through using timing. Plus, intermittent fasting has a variety of different options to fit different lifestyles and needs. In short, intermittent fasting is for you!

If you are ready for your best body and the best health of your life, then read on. This guidebook has everything you need to know about intermittent fasting, including how to do it, how to prepare for it, how to mitigate the possible side effects of doing it, and how to improve outcomes of cardiovascular disease and Type 2 Diabetes using its methods. This guide answers many questions you may have about this way of eating.

There are countless books on the market on this subject. It is great that you chose this one because this one is tailored to provide you the most options and the most honest examination of look at this way of eating. You will find out if the diet is for you and exactly how to use it in clear, concise chapters that will illuminate everything. You will find chapters about using intermittent fasting with diabetes and the ketogenic diet.

Don't put your health and your self-esteem on hold any longer. Jump in and learn how to have the best body of your life via intermittent fasting. You will be so glad that you did!

Chapter 1 - What is Intermittent Fasting?

Let's start by clearing up some common misconceptions about what intermittent fasting is so that you know into what you are getting.

What Fasting is Not

Intermittent fasting is not the same as starving yourself. Starvation is a severe deficit in caloric intake, resulting is not enough nutrition for your cells to operate. Starvation causes irreversible organ damage, brain fog, and even death. The epidemic of women suffering from anorexia shows how starvation leads to poor performance and eventual hospitalization and death. You do not want to starve yourself ever, and intermittent fasting does not call for starvation.

Fasting is diametrically opposed to starvation. The words are often used interchangeably. They should not be. Fasting is using control over your diet, and when you eat, giving you the ultimate control over your nutrition and your body. Starvation is uncontrolled and calls for long periods of not eating, which inevitably lead to either hospitalization or long periods of binging because the body desperately tries to make up for the nutritional deficiencies it has experienced. People who are starving without choice are miserable; turn on the TV, and you can see children holding bowls, begging for food with their ribs sticking out. They don't have a choice, and their bodies are paying for it. You have a choice, and you should not do this torture to your body.

So, What is Fasting?

The Independent believes that intermittent fasting became so popular with Jennifer Aniston and Miranda Kerr. Aniston starved herself skinny for the role of Rachel on *Friends,* making other women envy her tiny waist and chicken wing shoulder-blades. Miranda Kerr made people jealous as she strutted in beautiful dresses with Orlando Bloom on her arm. The popularity of starvation in Hollywood is, however, hardly new. It can be traced back to a model named Twiggy, who created the trend for models to be rail thin. It is no secret that Hollywood is a hotbed of fad diets, many of which are unhealthy. These stars then show off their thin bodies and make non-celebrities think, "I want to look like that."

A healthier approach can be observed in the Silicon Valley, where some of the biggest IT geniuses can be seen using intermittent fasting. These people are more concerned about computers than looking sexy for roles on TV or modeling gigs, so why do they do it? The answer is that they have uncovered a secret: intermittent fasting helps them keep their brains sharper.

So much so, that leaders of many high-tech companies organize group hunger strikes among employees. For instance, there is a Silicon Valley group called WeFa.st with monthly meetings and online groups where members of Slack and Facebook share tips for successful fasting [1]. This group is one of many that shows a striking move toward fasting as a way of eating among tech stars and gurus.

A Japanese biologist named Yoshinori Ohsumi received the Nobel Prize in 2016 for his studies on autophagy, or cellular self-eating, in Baker's yeast that was fasting [2]. In autophagy, the scientist proved that the body "cleans itself up" during fasting. The body will dispose of old cells and cellular debris in normal human waste during this period [2]. This process can counteract the negative effects of aging as well as illnesses such as cancer. Using this research, Silicone Valley greats began to try to defeat aging by improving their mental sharpness through fasting. They are not starving themselves, but rather doing something to improve their health by limiting what and when they eat.

To break it down, fasting is simply the time between when you finish the last meal of the day and start your first meal of the morning. Most people already naturally fast overnight between dinner and breakfast. The minute you sink your teeth into some toast in the morning, you break your fast, hence the name "breakfast." Some people may call any time between meals fasting.

Some people fast for religious reasons. They abstain from food during certain times of the day or for a period of days. There is no real duration for fasting. However, the optimal duration of fasting for improved health will be covered in later chapters.

Fasting is not starving yourself; it is taking a break from eating to let your body renew itself.

What is Intermittent Fasting?

Intermittent fasting [IF] is a planned form of fasting that lasts for a set duration, usually cyclically. You set a schedule for eating and stick to it. You may also have a specific diet that you follow during your eating windows or the times when you are not fasting. All of these logistics will be discussed in Chapter 5.

How do you know if intermittent fasting works? You will discover thousands of people with anecdotal evidence that it works wonders to improve your mental focus and clarity, fitness, and weight. However, few clinical studies have been completed on this approach. Many studies which have focused on low-calorie diets have observed some positive health impacts of fasting, but not enough has been studied on eating normal, safe amounts of calories during specific eating windows. Only one study by the US National Institute of Health has officially declared similarities between intermittent fasting and low-calories diets [3].

Basically, this study's findings suggest that intermittent fasting and low-calories dieting put stress on cells without causing them harm [3]. They increase insulin sensitivity and reduce blood glucose levels. They also cause insulin levels to drop, which decreases your body's desire to store fat. Animals subjected to intermittent fasting had superior leaning abilities, memory, reduced oxidative stress (which causes your cells to age), and improved immunity to disease [3]. Mattson hypothesized that putting the body through the stress of fasting allows the cells to adapt to the stress, which helps them fight off disease more successfully [3].

Further studies show that the body begins to eat its own fat stores after just ten to sixteen hours of fasting. The body will lose weight if a person combines intermittent fasting and low-calorie eating during their eating windows [4].

Chapter 2 - Science Behind Intermittent Fasting

As you have already read, the 2016 Nobel Prize went to Yoshinori Ohsumi for his work on autophagy. He also got the Breakthrough Prize in 2017 for the same research. As a professor at the Tokyo Institute of Technology's Institute of Innovative Research, he is an authority on how autophagy works.

Autophagy: The Cellular Garbage Man

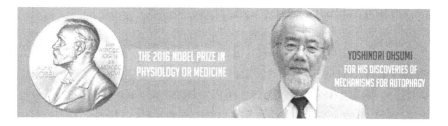

Autophagocytosis (autophagy for short) comes from the Greek words "autophagos," meaning "self-devouring," and "kytos," meaning "hollow." Basically, it illustrates how the cell will destroy parts of itself that are no longer optimal. Dr. Fung discusses how this process is essential for your body to eliminate aging and dysfunctional or even diseased cells and cell parts to keep your body running optimally. Think of your body like an engine. If one part is not running as well as the rest, it drains energy from the rest of the engine, causing the car's performance to suffer. You wouldn't think twice about replacing that part of the engine. So why not let your body do its job and replace its old cellular parts?

Basically, when we fast, our body has a chance to renew small parts of itself. The body will run out of glycogen, or sugar stores, and be forced to run on its fat stores instead. The result is that you lose fat. But to release the fat in your body's fat stores, insulin is required. Insulin is the critical hormone that basically unlocks cells to enable them to receive nutrition in the form of glucose from the bloodstream. Diabetes is a disease where, somehow, insulin is not being produced, or the cells are not receiving the glucose, causing them not to absorb nutrition from the blood.

To enter autophagy, your insulin level must drop low. Insulin will drop low if you don't eat for a while because it has no glucose in the cells to metabolize. This part of the process tells you that you're hungry. As a result, you eat and insulin spikes back up to "cover" the new flood of nutrition in your body. Your body stops tapping into its fat stores and uses the glucose that the food you ate provided since it is a readier form of energy. However, if you don't eat when you feel hungry, your insulin level stays low. Then your body begins to eat its fat again, and you can lose weight. Intermittent fasting allows you to accomplish this place where the body eats fat.

But there is more to intermittent fasting than just losing fat. The body's ability to clean itself out is exacerbated by intermittent fasting. The body can get rid of cells that may be turning cancerous, or that may lead to dementia, which is the real reason that Ohsumi won the Nobel Prize. He figured out that autophagy lets the body heal itself by getting rid of bad cells, reducing cancer and dementia risks, or fighting these diseases if they are already present in the body.

Autophagy is a method for the body to get rid of useless cells and organelles and proteins. You can harness this process with intermittent fasting. Lose weight, fight cancer and dementia, cleanse out toxins, and control insulin by simply fasting during set periods.

Chapter 3 - Health Benefits, Cautions, and Myths of Intermittent Fasting

The Numerous Health Benefits

As you can see, IF brings a host of health benefits along with weight loss. This striking difference is not starvation, which strips your body of nutrients and eventually leads to death. Obviously, there are more reasons than one to try intermittent fasting.

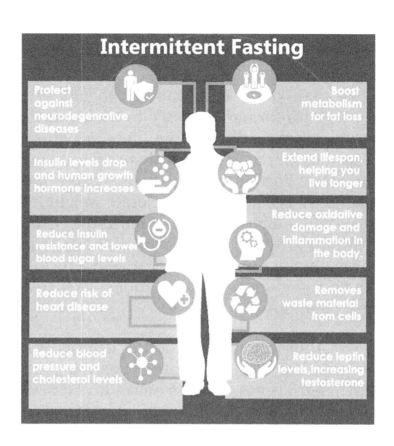

Healthier Way to Lose Weight

Fad diets tend to use bogus (or partially accurate) information to try to trick your body into losing weight. While some diets are supported by research, they are notoriously restrictive and hard to maintain. Furthermore, they may cause more harm than good because they accelerate weight loss. If you keep yo-yo dieting, you are more likely to get sick. Out of a group of 3,700 people, those who had the most fluctuations of weight tended to die the soonest and have complications like strokes and heart issues [6].

Intermittent fasting is a healthy way to lose weight. You lose weight by eating well during restricted times. There are no crazy dietary restrictions. You should not just gorge on junk food during your eating window, but you have a lot of liberty to choose what you eat. Then you let your body rest and go into the autophagic mode, which rejuvenates your cells. Through this method, you gain health rather than weight.

Intermittent fasting also shrinks your stomach naturally, much the way gastric bypass surgery does. You feel fuller faster and don't overeat. Also, IF ensures you drink enough water. You learn to drink water when you feel hungry, which is often mistaken thirst.

Last but not least, IF enables you to learn the self-discipline that can keep the weight off. It is not just some fad diet that you eventually end. It becomes a life-long habit that rewards you for the longer you do it.

It Is More Convenient

IF is easy to do. Its convenience makes it possible for any busy person. Think about it: There is no need to stop for food or prep meals or count calories during your fasting window. During your eating window, you can eat normally. You don't need to spend hours preparing food you don't like, nor do you need to buy into some program.

All you have to do is watch the clock to keep track of when you ate last. A written form or diary may not be necessary if you can remember it. Even a phone reminder is sufficient to keep track of your fasting cycles. There are phone apps designed for that purpose, some are for free, and some other apps charge money. Don't eat during certain times and eat at other times. It is that simple.

The ability to customize fasting is great too. You can work fasts around big events where you have to eat. Say, Thanksgiving is coming. You can plan your eating window around the family dinner and then fast at a different time for the rest of the day. Or if you find that you enjoy breakfast, plan your eating window around your usual breakfast time and fast at other times. You can even adjust your fast if you cheat – say you eat an hour early, just move your fast an hour later.

You Can Eat What You Want

IF does not come with a huge book of recipes for a reason: there are no steadfast rules beyond eating within certain time frames and fasting during the rest of the day. You will find that eating healthily during your eating window may, however, aid in weight loss and general well-being. It is always advisable to try to eat well instead of eating junk constantly.

However, if you want a hunk of cake at your friend's party, go for it. You do not have to feel guilty or count calories. You can enjoy the foods you want during the time frame you have selected for your eating window.

Eating Out Is Still a Breeze

Do you still want to eat out? That's fine. You don't need to bring a little container of carrots and abstain from the delicious dishes everyone else is enjoying. Have a craving for Chinese food? That's great, order some, because you can eat it. This diet will not get in the way of dates, family outings, or office parties at restaurants. You can even stop and get fast food occasionally, though of course it is not recommended that you eat excessive amounts of fast food. IF will not impede your favorite foods or eating out in any way. You have to plan for it and fit it into your fasting cycle.

Prevents You From Overeating

The longer you are on IF, the smaller amount you will want to eat. This situation does not mean that you will ever want to starve – your body demands nourishment, and it will eat what it needs. But we as a nation are programmed to overeat and think that we need a certain number of meals a day. That's why we tend to stuff our faces when we have already met our caloric requirement for the day. IF trains you to stop thinking this way and to feel full when you have reached nourishment. You will not want to overeat anymore because your body is used to not eating and can tell when it is full. Your new found self-discipline will also prevent you from overeating.

No More Need for Dangerous Diets

Those weird diets that have you eat a hard-boiled egg for breakfast and black coffee for lunch are not only dull and unpleasant but dangerous. They are not backed by sound scientific research confirming that they are safe. Ask your doctor, and he will tell you that most of these fad diets are far from healthy.

Now you don't need to buy whole books and workout DVD programs that you only use for a week. You don't have to follow weird Instagram diet challenges that make you hate life. Above all, you don't have to sacrifice your health for the sake of dieting. IF will do all of the fat burning for you, without weird dietary rules.

Reduces Inflammation And Physical Stress

Inflammation often drives pain and other chronic diseases. When your tissues are inflamed, they are not functioning at optimal capacity. This inflammation results in a lot of health problems. But IF has been shown to reduce this problem [8]. By reducing inflammation, You can see how it would help the pain.

Sugar is the number one cause of inflammation. By fasting and letting your insulin level out, you remove sugar from your body and burn fat instead. This step results in reduced inflammation and the health issues that come along with it.

Boosts Your Immune System

IF can help you to heal faster and fight off diseases more easily. As your body rests from digestion during fasting and begins cellular clean-up, it is better able to devote its energy to healing injuries and illnesses. People who fast report fewer illnesses and common colds.

Prevents Chronic Diseases

Better yet, there is evidence that IF can prevent heart disease and cancer [1]. By removing oxidative stress from the cells, the body is better able to remove damaged or mutated cells that could go on to cause cancer or Alzheimer's. It can also reduce inflammation related to illnesses like endometriosis, rheumatoid arthritis, and other painful diseases. All of these factors mean that IF can successfully reduce symptoms or even prevent chronic diseases.

May Extend Your Lifespan

With all of these great health benefits, it only follows that IF is good for longevity. With fewer illnesses and less aging, your life span may increase. You may also enjoy more quality of life as you age.

Increased Ketones

As anyone who has ever tried the ketogenic diet, you know that ketones single out fat loss. What happens is that ketones are the acids produced after your body burns its own fat. It starts to burn its own fat when it doesn't have sugar to burn. By going for long periods without sugar, your body begins to dip into its fat stores. A blood or urine test will indicate positive ketones, meaning your body is in ketosis or fat-burning mode.

Boosts Growth Hormone Production

HGH, or human growth hormone, was shown to increase five-fold in athletes who tried IF [7] leading to greater muscle growth. As you fast, you don't lose muscle mass, as you do with many dangerous diets. Rather, you lose actual fat and stimulate muscle growth. You can also increase stamina and endurance for working out.

Prevents Insulin Resistance

As you eat, your body produces more and more insulin to help absorb the food. Alternatively, if you are a diabetic, you must take more insulin injections to cover what you eat. By going without eating for some time, you create less insulin. This practice makes your cells less "used to it," causing insulin sensitivity to go up, which can reverse Type 2 diabetes.

It is not a good thing to have lots of insulin in your blood. Insulin triggers your body to hold onto fat, and fat cells are insulin resistant. The result is that you need yet more insulin to control your blood glucose. That process makes more fat. You can see the vicious cycle here, as it wreaks havoc on your body. Insulin resistance causes both weight gain and insulin resistance. The only way to reverse it is to lower the amount of insulin available in the body. Non-diabetics can do this by eating less. insulin-dependent diabetics can do this by simply eating less. It requires fewer shots or doses of bolus insulin.

Stable Glucose Levels

Another benefit of increased insulin sensitivity and less insulin in your body is stable blood glucose levels. As you stop requiring so much insulin, you are less prone to spikes and then drops as the sugar in your blood runs out and the insulin is still left behind.

Low blood glucose, or hypoglycemia, can affect non-diabetics and non-hypoglycemics. Your blood glucose may not be dangerously low, but you can still feel it. You feel weak, dizzy, and even nauseous. You go into panic attacks or snap at other people for no reason. You end the day with a terrible headache and have to lay down. Your energy is zapped, and your mood is bad. All of these things are a sign that your sugar has crashed. The natural instinct is to eat more sugar, but that only starts the cycle over again.

Non-diabetics will never experience high blood glucose in normal circumstances. However, having lots of sugar in your body calls for lots of insulin. Sugar is essentially a fast-burning fuel, so it goes fast. Then there is lingering insulin after eating lots of sugar, the crash is inevitable.

Instead, you can use IF to stabilize blood sugars. You avoid excess sugar, and you don't eat for periods, during which your body can stabilize itself by reducing insulin output. With no need for insulin, the body won't produce it. Your body falls into a cyclical harmony with your eating and fasting windows.

Reducing the Stress Hormone Levels

Cortisol is another sneaky hormone that leads to weight gain. When you are stressed, you tend to have a lot of cortisol running through your body. The cortisol tells your body that something bad is about to happen, so your body stores fat for energy. If you aren't running from a lion, however, you don't need this stored energy. It turns to the fat that you wear for the rest of your life unless you do something about it. IF can help you deal with stress better by exposing your cells to more stress [1]. They become better at handling the stress they experience and, thus, you react to life situations with less cortisol production.

Keeping Your Liver Healthy

Your liver is the main organ in your body that cleanses out toxins. By allowing your body to run autophagy during fasting, you make the load lighter on your liver. A fast will always cleanse your liver.

Intermittent Fasting is The Best Anti-Aging Agent

IF puts stress on your cells, which triggers them to "clean out" in autophagy. Oxidative stress is removed. Oxidative stress is normal wear and tear on cells that happens as you age.

Chemicals called free radicals run rampant in the world and your body [8]. These free radicals find the DNA proteins in your cells, and react with it, degrading it [9]. Over time, this can result in aged, unhealthy cells. But autophagy lets the body identify and remove these damaged cells [9].

Reduces the Risk of Heart Diseases

Heart disease is no joke. It is the number one killer of Americans, but you can almost completely halt its progression or prevent it altogether with intermittent fasting. It lowers blood pressure, the cholesterol, and triglycerides in the blood, improving your blood flow and putting less stress on your heart [10]. Lower levels of these elements mean better cardiovascular health.

Cautions

Like all diets, there are some things you must watch for while using intermittent fasting. You cannot reasonably expect to implement this way of eating without some sort of changes to your body. While fasting is not dangerous, you should watch to make sure your body is handling the adjustment.

Children

Children are still growing and need adequate nutrition more than ever. IF can deprive a child of valuable nutrition. It is never appropriate to start a child on such a diet unless supervised and approved by your pediatrician.

Pregnancy and Breastfeeding

Under no circumstances should a woman perform IF while pregnant or breastfeeding. Ask your doctor before you fast, if you are trying to conceive or just had a baby. The body's needs change with pregnancy and breastfeeding, and IF can be dangerous during these times.

You Might Struggle to Maintain Blood Sugar Levels

Especially for diabetics, blood sugar levels may drop too low. You must talk to your doctor if you cannot sustain healthy blood sugar levels. While the point of IF is to drop your blood glucose, it should not drop it below 80 mg/dl. Going too low can cause fainting or even coma or death, as well as heart and brain issues. Therefore, avoid IF in the event that it causes these issues, or eat more in your eating windows. if you take insulin, always only lower with the supervision of your doctor. Diabetics may want to consume juice if they drop too low. While this procedure breaks the fast, it will prevent dangerous hypoglycemic episodes that can be lethal. You can safely resume the fast once your blood glucose is back to normal if your doctor approves.

You Might Experience Hormonal Imbalances

If you do IF wrong, you create starvation, when you don't get sufficient nutrients. This situation goes beyond calories to include vital vitamins and minerals. Creating starvation can lead to hormone imbalances.

You Might Get Cravings

Until your brain learns to cope with the strenuous task of resisting food when it's used to eating, you may get strong cravings. You want something with all of your might. Drinking bone broth or black coffee can suppress your appetite and help you feel better. You may also try herbal tea with appetite suppressant properties, like peppermint tea.

You Might Get Headaches

Headaches from IF are typically dull and throbbing. They will pass with time. They are caused by the stress of the change as well as lower blood sugar levels. To fight them, try drinking more water and do relaxation breathing exercises. This symptom should go away in a few weeks.

You Might Experience Low Energy And Irritability

Often this irritability and fatigue are caused by low sodium and electrolytes. Drink Gatorade or bone broth. It will enliven you a bit. Also, increase your water intake for more energy and pep.

Use a journal to work through your feelings of irritability instead of taking them out on others or giving up on fasting. If you take the time to write it out, you might see that you are really not mad about anything at all.

You Might Experience Heartburn, Bloating, or Constipation

These are common ailments for those who are in fasting. Heartburn is often the result of stomach acid entering your esophagus, and it will pass as your body chemistry adjusts to the new eating schedule. Just drink more water and sleep with pillows propped under your upper back to keep the acid down. Also, try to avoid stress.

Bloating is typically caused by water retention from constipation. Drink lots of water. You can also try an over-the-counter water pill.

To treat constipation, try eating less fiber and drinking more water. Too much fiber can make your stools too hard and dry to pass.

If you have diarrhea, increase your fiber. Eat some fiber bars or more leafy greens and oatmeal. Fiber helps solidify your stools by holding onto water. Loose water in your bowels can cause loose stools. Persistent diarrhea, especially when coupled with blood, or fever or vomiting, warrants a trip to the ER because these symptoms are not caused by fasting but rather some other illness or infection.

You Might Start Feeling Cold

Coldness is a very common complaint of those doing IF. The coldness is caused by a decrease in sugar in your body. Sugar burns hot, so to speak, and it increases inflammation. It makes you feel warmer. Without it, your sensitivity to cold will increase. This symptom does not mean that you are cold – it simply means you respond more sharply to the environmental cold around you. Get a nice sweater and bundle up or sit in the sun for some extra vitamin D.

You Might Find Yourself Overeating

The major downside to IF is that not everyone has the self-control to do it. This point does not mean that you should give up in the event that IF makes you lose control and overeat during your eating window, or even break down and eat when you should be fasting. It t means you may need to switch programs and try one that calls for fasting when you are sleeping or busy at work. If you stay busy or asleep and are distracted from hunger, you won't want to overeat as much. You also can prevent overeating by eating more filling meals packed with fiber and protein during your eating windows.

You Might Have To Go To the Bathroom...a Lot

Autophagy is a process of cellular clean-up, meaning that your body produces more waste when it is going on in full mode. During IF, you may have to use the bathroom a lot to expel this waste. The diet may also make you drink more water, causing you to need to do number one more often. Many people have reported diarrhea when they start IF.

Common Myths About Intermittent Fasting

There are so many myths about intermittent fasting circulating in health books and on the Internet. These erroneous statements have created a stigma around intermittent fasting that causes people to avoid following this breakthrough diet. Learn to see through these myths which are not true.

Fasting is Dangerous

This first myth is simply ridiculous. Everyone intermittently fasts as they sleep. Doing it at other times or for a few days on end is no more dangerous than simply fasting while you sleep. The body needs a period to perform autophagy, and it cannot do that if it is too busy processing food all of the time. Intermittent fasting gives your body a well-deserved break while helping you preserve your health.

Remember, fasting is not starvation. You can still eat. Don't confuse fasting, which is healthful with starvation, which is dangerous.

Fasting Can Lower Your Blood Sugar Dangerously

The body can maintain its own blood glucose levels by releasing glycogen, or sugar stored in the liver [1]. This fact means that you won't go low dangerously if you stop eating for a spell. Instead, it will balance out and cause your body to start burning fat. The fat will keep you nourished and prevent fainting from not eating.

If you feel faint or lightheaded, you may need to eat. Be sure to listen to your body. Decrease your fasting period if you keep having dizzy spells.

However, if you are diabetic or hypoglycemic, you may need some help to maintain blood sugars during fasting. Ask your doctor how you can do this maintenance. Some fruit juice will technically break your fast, but it is necessary if your blood glucose plummets down.

It Will Cause Hormonal Imbalance

If anything, IF will balance your hormones. Doing IF wrong will indeed cause leptin and ghrelin, the main hunger hormones, to go crazy and make people binge [11]. Then they will feel guilty and restrict themselves more [11]. The hormones will get even more imbalanced. This effect can suppress a woman's ovulation and even stop her period [11]. However, a woman who implements IF correctly by keeping herself nourished in her eating windows will not experience this at all.

It Will Destroy Your Metabolism

Your metabolism will run on whatever energy source is easiest. Sugar from food is the easiest, so your body burns that first. With no sugar present, the body turns to burn its own fat cells. Either way, your metabolism works. You cannot destroy it.

Some say that if you fast, you will overeat and then have even more trouble losing the weight. This problem is psychological, not physiological. Often people hate restrictive diets so much that they do overeat when they stop dieting, causing them to gain the weight back. Then, they are resistant to new diet approaches and have trouble losing the regained weight. Affecting over 80% of people who have dieted, this problem is pretty common. But if you stick with IF and nourish yourself properly, you won't return to overeating, and you won't have this problem. IF doesn't ruin your metabolism to the point where you can't lose weight again if you do gain any back.

It Causes Stress

Technically, fasting is a period of stress. But as Dr. Fung points out, it is good stress that causes your cells to do their work more efficiently and handle the stress of illness more successfully [2]. Therefore, fasting will not cause extra stress.

The first week or so can be stressful because the approach involves change. Relax a lot and do things you enjoy or find soothing. The stress will pass.

Fasting Can Lead to Overeating

If executed with care, you can avoid the urge to binge eat later. It is true that fasting will make you hungry because of your body's hunger signals. You may feel the urge to eat more when you can or cheat on your fast. The key here is to keep yourself well- nourished when you do eat. Use bone broth to stave off cravings during fasting periods. Also, avoid going on long fasts when you first start. Don't allow the temptation of food around you or have lots of easy snacks in the house as you fast.

Fasting Causes the Body to go into Starvation Mode

Starvation mode is a myth that some people believe causes the body to hold onto weight when it perceives that it is not getting sufficient calories. Look at any person who has starved themselves, and you will see rapid, immediate weight loss and wasting. That picture of starvation proves that restricting calories to dangerous levels will not cause weight gain, but rather weight loss. Plus, fasting is not a dangerous caloric restriction or starvation so it will not cause any unhealthy "mode."

Fasting Causes the Body to Burn Muscle

Because fasting stimulates the production of HGH, it builds muscle rather than destroys it. It only promotes your body to eat fat, not muscle. People tend to start losing muscle mass if they consume too few calories, or essentially starve themselves. But they will not lose muscle if they stay nourished and hydrated and eat well between fasting periods.

You Can't Work Out While Fasting

You can absolutely work out while fasting. If you have eaten well during your eating window and have some extra body fat, exercise will only make your body burn more. Your body will get the nutrition it needs to fuel the workout from your fat stores and the last meal you ate. Be sure to stay hydrated for energy.

Chapter 4 – The Bare Bones of Intermittent Fasting

Here it is, the basics on how to implement this diet. You will need to read this chapter carefully to learn how to implement intermittent fasting safely and wisely.

How Long

How long you can fast is really up to you. Your body may not handle a long fast at first because it is not used to it. It will freak out, and you will not know how to respond to hunger pangs. As a result, you will break your fast before you are meant to and minimize results. Start small and make your fasts longer as you feel ready.

It is possible to fast for several days without issues. But if you feel lightheaded, you may need to break your fast. This lightheadedness is typically a symptom of low blood glucose, meaning your body is not able to sustain itself anymore.

Read on to learn about the different types of fasting and how they work. Be sure to pick the one that works for your schedule. You may not want to be fasting on a weekend when your family has a barbecue, for instance. Or if you have dinner with your family every night, be sure to pick a fast that allows having an eating window during dinner. Customize fasts so that they work for you. That is how to be successful in this approach. Otherwise, you will get frustrated and quit if you pick a fast that is too hard for you or that cuts into your life too much.

Types of Intermittent Fasting

There are several types of intermittent fasting available to fit your schedule and needs. It is often advisable to start with a small fast, such as 12 hours, to get your body used to it and to learn to ignore hunger pangs. Once you have mastered that, you can move onto a new system that calls for longer periods between eating windows. Taking baby steps helps you master the self-discipline and control that is so essential in this way of eating.

12-Hour Fast

In this simple fast, which is recommended for beginners, you fast for twelve hours and eat for twelve hours. So basically, you split your day in half. It is easiest to fast while you sleep and the few hours before going to bed and after you wake up. You will repeat this every day of the week.

16:8 Fasting

16:8 involves fasting for sixteen hours and then eating during eight. It is recommended to time breakfast around lunch and then stop eating after dinner so that you sleep through most of the fast. You will repeat this every day of the week.

5:2 Fasting

AKA the Fast Diet, 5:2 is a little bit different. In this diet, you don't ever have not to eat. You instead spend five days eating your normal number of calories. Then you spend two, preferably back to back, eating only 500-600 calories.

Alternating Days

You eat normally one day and don't eat the next. You fast every other day and eat every other day, so the days alternate. This plan is great because it gives your body 24 hours to rest and cleanse, and 24 hours to fuel up. It eliminates the math of figuring out when your next meal should be, as well. For those who are new to fasting or who cannot completely abstain from food, you can cut down to 500 calories on your fasting day and eat normally on your non-fasting day.

The con is that you can seriously overeat or fail to learn the self-control to honor your fast. You can also have more trouble planning fasts around important events if said event happens to fall on the day you are supposed to be fasting.

24 Hour Weekly Fasting (Up Day/ Down Day Fasting or the Eat-Stop Diet)

In this fasting protocol, you only fast for 24 hours once a week. The other six days are normal eating days. Your fast will begin with breakfast or lunch one day and extend to breakfast or lunch the next. It is great for weekends, or hectic work days when you will be too busy to eat anyway.

The pro is that you don't have to make fasting a big deal because you only do it once a week. The con is that you can forget that day or lose the self-control and discipline to avoid eating for one day because you have programmed your mind to expect meals every day.

Meal Skipping

Meal skipping is simple. You don't eat breakfast, for instance. While people famously advise against meal skipping, there is really no harm in it. As you already know, fasting is not harmful, and missing one meal will not kill you. Find the meal you like the least and skip it. Just don't overeat on the other meals.

20/4 (The Warrior Diet) - One Meal A Day- (OMAD) - Warrior Diet Fasting

On the Warrior diet, you eat very little for 20 hours. Vegetables are allowed, as are things like bone broth. Heavy foods, like bread, meat, or potatoes, are absolutely not allowed. Then, for about four hours late in the day, you can eat a huge dinner of healthy fats, proteins, and vegetables. A pot roast would be a good option on this diet.

The pro is that this diet works with the body's natural Circadian rhythm. But the problem is that people may not consume enough calories or build enough fasting control. You may be driven to snack throughout the day.

Lean-Gains Method (14:10 Fasting)

In this method, you eat during ten hours of the day, say from 8 am to 6 pm. Then you fast the other fourteen hours. This fasting schedule is most like how people eat anyway and can be a great way to start fasting.

36 Hour Fast

This longer fast is where you don't eat for 36 hours straight before resuming your normal eating habits. You may perform this fast only once a month or whenever you feel it is best. You will eat dinner at 6 pm and then not eat anything the next day, and then you will eat breakfast at 6 am on the third day.

People should work up to these longer fasts. Doing fasts too quickly can cause your self-discipline to crumble and force you to give into hunger. It can also increase symptoms, although it does double benefits as well. Work on shorter fasts before you attempt this one. If you don't feel well during the fast, stop. Have your doctor's supervision if you are on any medication or insulin.

Women have been shown to have the most trouble with these longer fasts. The problem is that women have more sensitive hunger hormones and may binge after a longer fast, regaining weight they lost during the fast [11].

42 Hours

This plan works just like the 36-hour fast, except there are six more hours of fasting involved. Again, the same precautions should be used as with the 36-hour fast. In this case, you would eat dinner at 6 pm on Day 1, skip all meals on Day 2, and eat lunch at noon on Day 3.

During your eating window, do not restrict calories. That approach can be dangerous. It is imperative that you eat your daily allotment of calories during your eating window. So, on Day 1 and Day 3, eat the normal number of calories you eat during your usual diet.

60 hours - The Himalayan Fasting Diet

The longest fast of all, the Himalayan Fasting Diet is sixty hours. That is over two days of fasting! Two and a half days, to be precise. You start fasting after dinner and wait until breakfast on Day 4. You may eat up to 500 calories on Days 2 and 3 if you want. These calories should be made up of high-fat, high-protein, low-carb foods like fatty fish and avocados.

This diet is superior to the others because it really kicks in autophagy after 48 hours of fasting when glycogen is wiped out, and ketosis starts. You can benefit the most from doing this fast periodically. However, the cons are that it is hard to sustain, and symptoms can set in very dramatically.

Longer Fasts - Risks and Benefits

The benefits of longer fasts are that they show better results in shorter windows of time.

While it might take a year before you see results from a 12-hour fast, you will see results from a 60-hour fast on the day that you complete the fast.

But these longer fasts are much harder to do if your mind is not yet trained to accept hunger and ignore cravings. You are far more likely to crash and then binge. You must work up to these longer fasts.

These longer fasts can also interfere with your lifestyle. If you go on a long fast once a month, you will find it harder to skip or work around major events where food is involved. You will be more tempted by food as well.

The symptoms also become stronger in these longer fasts. You will suffer from more constipation, cold, fatigue, headaches, and other unpleasant sensations. You will be hit with more cravings and hunger pangs. All of these things can make you want to give up on the fast. If you work up to it, however, these symptoms will be less noticeable, and you can work through them.

Chapter 5 – Ready, Set, GO!

So now you are sold. You want to do intermittent fasting! But first, you really need to check with your doctor. We cannot emphasize this point enough. Your doctor may see issues with your health that can prevent you from fasting safely.

If you get the all-clear, then it is time to pick your fasting plan.

Learn What Your Natural Eating Pattern Is

Before beginning the fast, keep a journal. Note when you eat, how much, and what you eat. Your pattern may seem random until you document it. After all, the human body tends to fall into certain routines.

Once you know your pattern, you can customize your fast to a greater degree. Say you are especially hungry in the morning when you wake up. That might be a good time for your eating window. Or say, you eat the most at dinner. That should be your eating window.

You may also consider events like holidays and barbecues. No one wants to have to miss out on

Thanksgiving because of a diet. You can certainly plan for these days ahead of time.

Start With an Easier Fast

First, start with an easy fast, such as an overnight 12-hour fast from 6 pm to 6 am, and a 12-hour eating window from 6 am to 6 pm. This schedule should fall into your normal pattern of eating, so your body does not feel deprived. You can focus on teaching your body to handle the fast by avoiding the temptation for late-night ice cream runs or midnight snacks or even very late dinners. Beyond a few slight adjustments, you will be sleeping, and you won't have to do much to keep the fast going.

Transition Slowly

After about two weeks on your first fasting plan, you can begin to transition into a harder and longer fast. Start with a 16-hour fast and an 8-hour eating window. Then move up to the Warrior Diet that is 20 hours of fasting with a four-hour eating window. You can try one of these fasts for a week and then try the other, or switch between the two. These two plans should get you accustomed to vigorous fasting and the way you feel when you fast. It lets you learn coping mechanisms and discipline.

Try the other fasting plans after you have gotten used to the 16-hour plan and the Warrior Diet. This approach allows you to find the one that works for you. Not everyone is the same. What works wonders for one person may fail miserably for you. If a plan makes you miserable, choose a new one. You are guaranteed to fail if you stick to a plan that is not pleasant or realistic for you.

You may also plateau at some point, where your weight starts to stay the same. In this case, switch plans. Clearly, the one you are on is not working. First, however, be sure to watch how much water you drink and what you eat during your eating windows. Not drinking enough can make you hold onto water weight while bingeing on fast food or sugar during your eating windows can cause blood glucose crashes that encourage you to hold onto weight. If you are eating well, drinking enough, and still not losing weight, it may be time to try a new fasting plan.

Protect Your Motivation

Part of dieting involves protecting your mind and your motivation. There is nothing as bad as meddling family and friends when you are on a diet. These people love you, but they are poorly informed about intermittent fasting. They will try to discourage you from your diet and scare you into abandoning it before you can even enjoy results.

The best way to avoid their discouragement is to keep your diet to yourself. Plan your fasting around family events so that you can eat in front of family and not have to explain why you are not eating if you are fasting when a family member wants you to eat spontaneously, state that you are just not hungry.

Start it before you tell them so that they see your results and realize that you are not starving yourself. If you drop ten pounds and look great, they will relent on telling you to drop the diet.

Your family and friends may not want to hear about the diet, anyway because they have their own lives and may not be ready to see you succeed. That is OK. You can enjoy your results without letting them drag you down.

It can be helpful to have a fasting buddy. A significant other, family member, or good friend who believes in fasting and wants to lose weight can be a huge motivator. If you don't have a buddy, find a local group or a Facebook group of like-minded people to motivate you and give you tips. You can also keep a journal to chart your progress and feelings as you get to know your body. A journal is often helpful for people trying to get on track with something new.

When you want to give in and eat during your fasting window, a journal can be your best friend. Write about why you want to give in. Did someone bring a tray of cupcakes to the office? Did you have a rough day, and emotional eating is your way of coping? Find out why you want to give in. Then find a solution that does not involve eating. You can learn a lot about yourself, such as why you overeat or what triggers you to break your fast. That helps you to learn to avoid such triggers or cope with them in other ways in the future. For instance, when you have a bad day, go exercise to burn off stress as opposed to stuffing your face with ice cream while watching TV.

Before and after pictures can also motivate you when you feel like giving up. Look back at old pictures of yourself and remember how desperately you wanted to change. Look at your goal weight, or some health goal, and compare progress. You are likely doing better than you think.

Learn to Listen To Your Body

Your body sends you clear signals about what it is experiencing. You will fail at your diet if you ignore its signals. Many of its signals are based on mental conditioning that causes you to abandon your diet. Learn to recognize these signals and ignore them.

Often, people feel the urge to eat when they are really thirsty. The body seems to confuse thirst and hunger signals in modern people. If you feel a craving to eat, try drinking some water instead. Black coffee can also give you energy and stifle hunger.

If your stomach growls, then it is empty. You will naturally want to eat. You have always been conditioned to keep your stomach full and to eat three square meals a day or more. In time, your stomach will learn to feel more satisfied and not push for you to eat when it is empty. Simply ignore the hung pangs and chew on something like celery to trick your brain into thinking that your body has been fed. Drink lots of water to fill your stomach, as well.

Be sure to stay busy. Now is the perfect time to throw yourself into your work or pick up that hobby you have been putting off. A distraction will keep you from fixating on your hunger and surrendering to hunger pangs during your fasting window.

If your symptoms get a bit more unpleasant, you may need to eat. A foggy brain, lightheadedness, and even fainting are signs that you must eat. Eat something small and resume your fast.

Never ignore pain. If you experience sharp pains anywhere in your body, including your stomach, it is time to visit the doctor. Intermittent fasting does not cause pain. Hunger pangs should not hurt immensely. Something else is clearly wrong if you experience severe pain.

Eat Healthy In Between

What you do during your eating window is just as important as not eating during your fasting windows. You want to make sure that you fill this window in a healthy way that nourishes and sustains your body with proper hydration and nutrition. Otherwise, you will not lose weight or improve your health, and the whole point of this diet is missed.

Always start your day with water. Drink at least eight glasses throughout the day, preferably up to a gallon. Water keeps your stomach full and aids your body in often urinating to flush out the waste it has generated with autophagy. Water is also refreshing and gives you energy when you feel tired or weak. If you get sick of water, use calorie-free water flavor powders, black tea, or black coffee.

Choose wholesome meals with lots of fiber. Fiber will also keep you feeling fuller for longer so that the hunger pangs during your fasting window are minimized. It is best to eat whole grains, whole vegetables, and at least one serving of protein during each meal. It is often recommended to eat a rainbow, meaning that you should have a variety of vegetables, fruits, and other foods of different colors. These colors represent the vitamins and minerals in the food that keeps your body healthy.

Make your eating window count. You will regret it and cave to hunger pangs if you miss eating during this time. Be sure to fill yourself with foods that make you feel fuller for longer periods. More on what foods to pick will be covered later.

Stay Warm

Some people report chills or feeling cold when fasting. Have a comfortable sweater and slippers to keep yourself warm. Try exercising. Some jumping jacks can really heat you up by getting your blood flowing. A warm cup of tea with some cinnamon or hot water with lemon can also help to warm you up.

Avoid Excessive Levels Of Sugar

Sugar leads to your insulin spiking to cover it. The result? A sugar crash that makes you tired, cranky, and anxious for more fuel. Eating sugar will cause you only to eat more sugar. The best thing to do on any diet is to avoid lots of sugar.

If you crave sweets, distract yourself. Don't cave to the craving! Also, avoid sugar substitutes or diet sodas, because these items trick your brain into thinking you have eaten something sweet. Your brain will release more insulin for the sugar it is expecting. When that sugar is not there, you experience a sugar crash which makes you crave sweets even more.

Know When to Quit

Quitting is the only way to fail. But if you absolutely must quit, then do so. Fasting is not meant to be unhealthy or unpleasant. If it is unhealthy or unpleasant, then it is not working for you. It may be time to quit if your doctor says so if you're losing too much weight, if you can't follow the plans, or if you experience other health problems.

When you quit, don't use quitting as an excuse to return to unhealthy eating habits. You must find a new way to eat that is still beneficial. Otherwise, you will continue to hold onto or even gain weight, and you will feel terrible. You will also continue to damage your organs with unhealthy foods and excess sugar. View your time with fasting as a learning experience for how to adjust your diet to keep yourself healthy.

Chapter 6 - What Can You Eat and Drink During Intermittent Fasting

When doing IF, Not eating is only half of the equation Consuming twenty cheeseburgers and a pizza during your eating window will only defeat your health and weight loss goals by causing you to consume more calories than you need. Even if you use IF, you still must watch calories and keep them within your safe recommended limit.

Most people can eat 2,000 calories a day, but that depends on your weight, height, age, and gender. Use a calories calculator to find out the safe number of calories for you to eat to either maintain weight or lose one or two pounds a week. Then focus on consuming this amount during your eating window, no more and no less.

What Can You Eat While Fasting?

Above all, when you are using IF, you must drink water. Water, water, water. You should get up to a gallon a day. It doesn't have to be plain. You can get fizzy water, or flavored water that has no calories, or even add lemon or lime or cucumber for a refreshing change. You can also stir in apple cider vinegar, which aids in weight loss. Himalayan salt gives you electrolytes, which can fight off fatigue when you first start fasting.

You can drink up to six cups of coffee a day. You can add creamer or sugar during your eating windows (though sugar is best avoided anyway!). During fasting times, you cannot add anything to your coffee. Tea is also OK. Caffeine is acceptable. You may find that adding fat to your coffee, such as coconut oil or butter, helps you to sustain for longer during your fasting periods. Don't put in artificial sweeteners, milk, honey, sugar, or any powdered creamer during your fasting period. Spices like cinnamon can replace your need for sugar.

Seek herbal teas that also act as appetite suppressants. Cinnamon and chamomile tea can work as appetite suppressants. So do peppermint, bitter melon, oolong, chai, and green teas. They can also lower your blood sugar, causing less insulin to course through your body, aiding in fat loss. Supplements that purport to help with weight loss can be helpful too, but be sure they are from a reputable source and have no calories. You can only add lemon or cinnamon to your tea during fast.

Bone broth is also great during your fast. It can help with lightheadedness without adding lots of calories. It also adds gelatin to your bones, helping with joint issues. A vegetable or meat broth will also work. Feel free to consume a lot of broth when you first start fasting to help your body acclimate to not eating. You can wean yourself off and fast fully when your body is more accustomed to it.

To make your own bone broth, use animal bones and grind them up with any of the following: bitter melon, ground flaxseed, herbs, Himalayan salt, carrots, shallots, onions, leafy greens, and vegetables. Using this approach with broth is not breaking your fast because you will not be eating the ingredients, but instead drinking the liquid, they produce from the grinding process.

What Should You Eat During Your Eating Window?

During your eating window, you can eat whatever you want really. But to improve your health, you should focus on whole foods and vegetables with lots of vitamins and minerals. Plus, you should avoid high amounts of sugar to avoid sugar crashes and cravings later on. Eating foods with tons of fiber will fill you up, helping you navigate your fasting period more easily with fewer hunger pangs. Protein will also give you the energy you usually get from sugar, enabling you to perform more fully.

- Asparagus
- Avocado
- Bell Peppers
- Broccoli
- Brussel Sprouts
- Beans
- Cabbage
- Carrots
- Cauliflower
- Celery
- Chicken
- Cucumber
- Fatty fish
- Grass-fed beef
- Green Beans

- Kefir
- Kimchi
- Leafy greens
- Mushrooms
- Nuts (Avoid peanuts and cashews, which have high carb counts.)
- Nut butters
- Oatmeal
- Quinoa
- Snow Peas
- Sauerkraut
- Tomatoes
- Zucchini

For extra fiber, eat flaxseeds or wheat germ in your meals. Try satisfying snacks, like slices of apple with nut butter or avocado with some cottage cheese. Get probiotics in yogurt, kimchi, kefir, sauerkraut, and other fermented foods to aid digestion.

The above list is hardly exhaustive. Many foods are available. Remember, IF is not a diet with food restrictions. It is merely a habitual time management approach to eating. Thus, you can eat whatever you want during your eating window. However, for optimal health and weight loss results, stick to foods with low carbs and low sugar.

Chapter 7 - Intermittent Fasting For Women

Can women fast? The short answer is yes, absolutely. The long answer is that pregnant and nursing women should never fast and women who do fast should watch for uncomfortable symptoms. If you don't feel right, visit the doctor and cease fasting. Your body will let you know if something is wrong.

Women and men both respond to fasting well. However, women tend to respond to longer fasts better simply because they have more experience dieting. Women will lose less weight than men in the first two weeks, but they will catch up in the next four to six weeks. Many women do not always shed pounds on IF, either, but rather they notice more muscle mass and a better fit for their clothes. The number on the scale is not an indicator of successful weight loss.

Women who fast also often report positive hormonal changes. They have fewer ugly period symptoms, less brain fog, elevated moods, and better sex lives, certainly a win for women! The fact that autophagy can repel cancer by cleaning out damaged and mutated cells can also help women to stave off breast, ovarian, and cervical cancer worries.

Obesity and Its Impact on Women

Obesity is obviously not good for anyone. But for women, it can be especially disastrous because of its effect on female hormones. Fat cells produce their own estrogen [12]. This estrogen can become excessive, preventing proper progesterone production and upsetting the HPG axis, a delicate balance between hormones and the pituitary gland and the ovaries that regulates a woman's hormones and reproductive ability, as well as her endocrinological systems and moods [12]. The result is that women will develop a hormonal imbalance called estrogen dominance, leading to issues like endometriosis, cysts, trouble ovulating, weight gain, trouble sleeping, poor mood control, irregular or absent periods, heavy periods, and trouble sustaining pregnancy [12].

Obesity also creates insulin resistance, which leads to more insulin production and more insulin resistance. The excess insulin triggers ghrelin and leptin, the hormones that stimulate hunger. The result is increased weight gain and a drive to eat more, that causes more weight gain. It is a vicious cycle, out of which many women struggle. IF can help with these issues by increasing insulin sensitivity and controlling hunger, while also removing the fat that produces too much estrogen.

The Crucial Role of Cholesterol in a Woman's Life

Studies suggest that women need cholesterol, a wax that coats the veins, even more than men do. Women use cholesterol to manufacture estrogen, progesterone, bile acids, and vitamin D [13]. While the last two elements are essential for every human being, the first two hormones are key to a woman's reproductive health. She will not be able to release eggs, ovulate, possibly get pregnant, and then stop menstruation and hold onto the fertilized egg without healthy cholesterol.

But because women need cholesterol, their bodies tend to make more of it and hold onto it more vigorously [13]. Most women have elevated cholesterol and high cholesterol after menopause. High cholesterol will clog arteries, leading to heart strain and eventual heart trouble. It can also lead to visceral fat, dangerous fat that coats the organs and prevents healthy organ functioning.

Why Autophagy And Protein Cycling Matter Especially For Women

For women, the processes of protein cycling and autophagy are particularly important. Why is that? Because women are at risk for more types of cancer, with which fasting can help. Women tend to hold onto fat, which is disruptive to their hormones.

Now let's talk about protein cycling. Your body cannot create its own protein, so it must obtain protein from food sources. Women especially need protein to help burn fat and support hormonal health [14]. Protein also satiates women, helping them to overcome the cravings that tend to destroy their ability to sustain fasting [14]. Thus, an ideal approach involves eating lots of protein during eating windows and then fasting for up to 24 hours. This approach results in significant fat loss of up to ten percent [14].

Hormonal Effect of Fasting on Women

Women have more of a hormone called kisspeptin, which makes them much more sensitive to fasting than men [15]. They may also have more cortisol, which negatively influences their sleep cycles. Both of these hormones can cause a disruption in the HPG Axis, which will adversely affect the production of estrogen and progesterone.

Therefore, women should start fasting lightly. Then they should try a gentler approach [15]. They should also exercise only lightly on their periods and on fasting days. These approaches will help reduce the possible bad side effects of IF. Generally, once women get used to fasting, they find that it helps them to balance hormones, sleep better, and handle stress so much better because it actually balances their HPG Axis.

A Gentle Fasting Solution For Women

The best approach to fasting for women is to fast for 24 hours once or twice a week, or in other words, use 5:2 fasting. Then on eating days, women should load up on healthy sources of protein from plants and animals and nuts.

Women should also ease into fasting. Start with a 12-hour fast, move to 16:8, then try 5:2. Be sure to have bone broth on hand for protein and craving satiation during fasting. Only exercise when you feel well enough to do so. Do not push your body. Lightly exercise on fasting days or on your period. On period days, you must consume at least 500 calories and be sure to eat lots of iron-rich foods.

Eating enough calories is very important. If the body goes into starvation, it will turn off reproduction first, and hormones can be disrupted for a long time or even permanently [14]. This situation is why anorexic women typically lose the ability to get pregnant. Thus, you absolutely must eat sufficient calories in your eating windows.

Symptoms You Should Watch For

Any symptom that is so troubling it interferes with your quality of life is an issue for women. You should stop fasting and see a doctor if you experience any of the following symptoms:

- Unusual pelvic pain
- Bleeding with sex
- Unusual tiredness
- Pale skin
- Hair loss
- Weight gain
- Extreme weight loss (more than two pounds a week)
- Rashes on the skin
- Amenorrhea (the absence of a period for three months)
- Unusually painful and/or heavy periods
- Migraines
- Dizziness
- Fainting
- Vomiting
- Severe stomach pain

During Menstruation

Fasting will disrupt a woman's cycle, plain and simple. For menstruating women, this can mean that you stop your period. This disruption is only temporary until the body starts getting the nutrition it needs again. It is a reflex reaction to stress, which is the natural byproduct of fasting. IF will eventually lead to greater hormonal balance in women, if proper diet is practiced during eating windows. There is usually an adjustment phase that can be more noticeable in women who have more obvious signs of hormones such as menstruation.

Some women who engage in IF will discover pale skin, hair loss, missed periods, early onset menopause, and other hormonal issues. These issues usually subside in a few months if IF is appropriately practiced. That means not starving yourself for days on end, listening to your body, and eating a well-balanced diet with sufficient calories when in your eating windows. It also calls for taking a good multivitamin and listening to your doctor.

Menstruation is simply the expulsion of blood when your body does not detect pregnancy. Fasting does not necessarily affect it. Anecdotally, many women report fewer cramps and lighter bleeding during their periods, if they fast. It is your choice if you want to fast during your period or not. Often, women feel hungrier during their periods so you can forego fasting if it feels most comfortable for you. If you do decide to fast, be sure to eat more iron-rich foods, such as spinach and beef, and focus on more protein when you are in your eating windows.

During Menopause

Few studies show whether or not menopausal women should actually fast. Dr. Becky Gillapsy conducted a meta-review of studies done on fasting, women's health, and even getting older [15]. The results she found are that women experience fasting no differently than men, even menopausal women.

Menopause often signals for the body to stop producing certain hormones, which can accelerate health problems and aging. Fasting can help the body mitigate these issues through autophagy. Higher risks of breast cancer are a problem that menopausal women face, which can be eliminated by IF. Alzheimer's can also be avoided.

Chapter 8 - Intermittent Fasting and Diabetes

Type 2 Diabetes is often caused by being overweight, which creates insulin resistance in the cells. What can you do to reverse it? Obviously, losing weight to improve insulin sensitivity. Losing weight can help you manage or even reverse Type 2 Diabetes with a minimum of issues. As you well know, IF can help with weight loss tremendously.

Weight Loss and Type 2

Intermittent Fasting can help you lose weight with diabetes, but it has to be performed under the close supervision of your doctor. Especially if you are on insulin injections or medications, this form of dieting may cause adverse effects. This fact is also true for Type 1 diabetics who want to use IF.

Type 1 is an autoimmune disorder where the insulin cells in the pancreas are attacked and no longer able to function [5]. This problem causes insulin deficiency, and injections are required. Type 2 is different. One's body makes the insulin, but the cells can't absorb it. Usually, this phenomenon is caused by lifestyle and diet. As one consumes too much sugar, his body produces too much insulin, which can lead to insulin resistance [5]. Then medications may be in order. Fat cells are also naturally insulin resistant, so having too many fat cells in the body (too high of a body fat percentage) can also lead to insulin resistance. Drinking a 2-liter Coke every day for years will indeed make you sick.

If a person is obese, he or she is either diabetic or at serious risk to become one. Diabetes brings with it kidney failure, heart disease, stroke, vision loss, painful neuropathy, and limb amputation. That's why weight loss is so crucial.

Is There a Cure for Diabetes?

There is no absolute cure for diabetes, but most people have found that losing weight can halt or even reverse Type 2 diabetes. There is currently no cure for Type 1 diabetes, but weight loss can prove beneficial for Type 1 as well because by raising sensitivity, it lowers the amount of artificial insulin they must inject daily.

There was no way to treat diabetes before the mid-1800s. Most people died at age 50 when most Type 2 diabetics are diagnosed. Type 1 children would die. Insulin came into the picture in the 1920s, which helped to extend the lives of Type 1 diabetics, but the technology did not make their quality of life similar to non-diabetics until the 1990s [16]. However, something happened in the mid-1800s to help Type 2s, which started appearing around this time because more food was readily available.

You can credit Apollinaire Bouchardat (1806-1886) with finding the first real cure for Type 2 diabetes. He discovered that soldiers in the Franco-Prussian War were expelling less sugar in their urine after periods of starvation [16]. Thus, he began to recommend a sugar-free diet for diabetics, which he described in De la Glycosurie ou Diabete Sucre (Glycosuria or Diabetes Mellitus). His diet is just like low-carb diets prescribed to diabetics now.

Now, diet and exercise are the two biggest components of curing Type 2. There are many successful diabetes reversal stories out there. Dr. Fung presses on the importance of restricting carbs and sugar. IF can also help the body reduce insulin resistance, combining periods of fasting and eating windows of low-carb, high-protein meals can be a game changer for Type 2 diabetics.

History of Type 2 Diabetes

Diabetes can be traced back to 1500 BCE, but it was never fully understood until the late 1800s and early 1900s [16]. The discovery of how to make insulin from pigs in the 1920s helped Type 1 diabetics to survive their diagnoses, which, to that time were fatal [16]. But for Type 2 diabetics, the cure has been clear since Apollinaire's work: diet and exercise can save the life of a Type 2 diabetic. However, this knowledge has been cyclically lost and found throughout the centuries. Food shortages remove the eminence of Type 2 diabetes, and it only becomes an issue again when food is readily available, and obesity rates skyrocket. Obviously, now, Type 2 diabetes is a huge issue.

Now that obesity rates have risen, so have rates for Type 2 diabetes. Most obese people develop or show warning signs for developing Type 2. Even children, who used not to have many instances of Type 2 diabetes, are starting to get it. The secret lies in our high-sugar, high-fat diets and sedentary lifestyles. This way of eating and not exercising is actually killing us.

What Happens When You Strictly Control Diet?

Most medical professionals believe that Type 2 is a chronic and progressive disease, meaning that there is no cure and it will only get worse with time. But many stories can be found of people overcoming diabetes by simply controlling their eating. Dr. Fung points out that recipients of bariatric surgery, which reduces the size of the stomach to restrict the amount of food one can eat, often improve their diabetes [5]. Dr. Fund even observed that there is less glucose in the urine of those who have their food restricted by this surgery. Death rates from diabetes declined rapidly in the two world wars when food was rationed. All of this evidence indicates that diabetes can be controlled or even eliminated by simply restricting food.

Restricting food through fasting is a good way to accomplish this goal. As you eat less, you lose weight. Then you can change the progression of diabetes within your body. However, always plan to eat less with the supervision of your doctor.

Chapter 9 - Intermittent Fasting on Keto Diet

Intermittent fasting and the ketogenic diet are often combined to produce stunning fat loss results. The thing about both ways of eating is that they restrict food in such a way that they promote ketosis or fat burning. They both offer similar health benefits, as well. If used together, they can result in significant fat loss.

How to Combine the Two

Combining keto and fasting is easy. The two methods of eating can work in harmony, turning your body into a sleek fat-burning machine. You pick a fasting plan that works for you from earlier in the book, and then you eat keto-friendly foods on your eating days or during your eating windows.

Possibly the best fasting plan while on keto is the 16:8 method, or the 5:2 method. You don't need to go on long fasts while also on keto since your body is already in ketosis from the keto diet plan.

You can use intermittent fasting to reach ketosis first before launching a keto diet. Cleanse your body on a fast, such as the Warrior Method. When you stop fasting, make sure your meals are ketogenic. You want your first meal to have lots of fat and then continue eating that way. Satiate cravings and prevent overeating during eating windows with low-carb snacks, such as almonds or carrots. Then work fasting into a cycle, balanced with days of keto eating. If you ever slip up on keto by eating too many carbs and leaving ketosis, you can get back into it by fasting for a few days again.

Before you begin this combination, find a keto calculator online for free and enter the appropriate information. You will learn how many carbohydrates, fats, proteins, and overall calories you need per day. You also want to factor in dietary fiber, which keto often neglects to mention. Most people should aim for 25-30 grams of fiber per day. Fiber is essential for your health and smooth, easy stools, which can become too fluid with the high-fat content of ketogenic foods. Fiber has carbs, but they are generally negligible and will not add to your carb allotment.

Once you know this information, you can plan meals that get you the proper amount of nutrients of each kind during your eating windows. You can use fasting time to plan these meals and prepare for them, keeping yourself busy. Just don't fall into the temptation of eating while you cook!

Benefits of the Keto Diet When You're Fasting

The main benefit of fasting on the keto diet is that you will accelerate results because you will enter ketosis faster. On the keto diet, you restrict carbs and focus on eating high-fat foods to make your body stop relying on sugar and burn fat instead. The presence of ketones in the blood or urine announces that ketosis has commenced. But it can take days and very stringent dietary control to enter ketosis on the keto diet. Since IF can trigger ketosis in a matter of days, versus weeks on ketosis, it allows for entering fat-burning mode more efficiently.

Plus, many people will find themselves out of ketosis if they slip even a tiny bit on their keto diet. A few too many blueberries or a single piece of toast can end ketosis, and then the person must start all over again to get back into it. Fasting when you slip up on keto can help you slide into ketosis again more rapidly.

The diet is simplified with a routine set by fasting, as well. You know exactly what you can eat and when. During your eating window, you should get your calculated rate of fat and protein macros and keep carbs under 20 grams per day. During fasting, you don't have to worry about what to eat at all. And yes, water and bone broth are highly useful on both keto and fasting so that you can use them throughout your diet.

The keto diet can be hard to sustain, especially if you love your pasta or donuts. So, since fasting is a way of eating that can become a lifelong habit, it can eventually replace keto and help you still keep the pounds off. You can use keto to get thin fast and then start using IF to keep thin in the future. There is no need to stay on keto forever if you don't like it.

The final and biggest benefit is that IF teaches you not to overeat and overcome cravings. Thus, it prepares your mind for the effort required to stick to the keto eating plan. It also enables you to ignore cravings and control your portions, staying within your macro limits on keto.

Side Effects of Fasting on the Keto Diet

The primary side effect of fasting while on the ketogenic diet involves the keto flu. The keto flu is a collection of nasty symptoms that arise in the first week or so of ketosis, which can be exacerbated by fasting.

Keto flu involves extreme fatigue, irritability, sore muscles, bad breath, feeling cold, and headaches. It can cause women to report smelly vaginal discharge. Usually, this flu goes away in a few days. To tolerate it, you should drink lots of electrolytes and increase your salt intake. Try eating a few days of keto before you try fasting to get over the symptoms naturally.

Of course, fainting, vomiting, hair loss, or extreme pain of any kind, are all worrisome symptoms. Stop your diet and fasting altogether, and get a blood workup at the hospital. Make sure you don't have a severe hormonal or mineral deficiency or any other serious health issues before you start the diet and fasting again.

The point of both keto and fasting is that your blood sugar is meant to go low. But if it goes too low, definitely talk to your doctor. If you are an insulin-dependent diabetic, you want especially to have your doctor's help to lower your insulin to prevent hypoglycemia.

Many people, particularly women, are prone to plateauing on keto. A fast can help to break that plateau. If your weight loss stalls and you still have not reached your goal weight, consider reevaluating how often you fast and take a longer fast. You might also consider lowering your caloric intake on eating days.

Things to Consider

You want to ensure that you get the appropriate number of calories.

The main issue with combining keto and fasting is that you may not get enough calories, and then you starve. Malnutrition is not the goal here, and it will not lead to healthy weight loss. It can cause hormonal imbalances, organ damage, brain damage, illness, muscle loss, metabolic slowdown, and other issues.

The great thing about fats is that they are filling. Therefore, eating keto meals in your eating windows will help you avoid hunger later on. But many people on keto fail to consider how much fat they are eating and they tend to skimp on the number of fat calories they require. They spend more time ensuring that they do not eat over twenty grams of carbohydrates, and they do not count fat. Going over or under on fat calories will defeat the diet, so be sure to use a keto calculator free online to find how many macros you need to consume each day. Factor that into your diet plan to avoid overeating, hunger, or loss of muscle mass.

Make sure you are getting adequate vitamins and minerals. A daily supplement is a good place to start, but often it doesn't have enough of every element, or it is not absorbed in your body thoroughly. Therefore, you must also get vitamins and minerals from the food you eat. Dairy from calcium, iron from kale or spinach, vitamin D from mushrooms, vitamin C, and beta carotene from carrots and bell peppers, and vitamin E from almonds are all great places to start. In moderation, berries are keto-friendly and contain vitamin C and antioxidants to prevent aging.

Chapter 10 - Intermittent Fasting Success Stories

If you have any doubts, then look to those who have tread before you. These stories are from real women who have lost weight using IF. Most people who try this way of eating are very happy with their results. Some people are mad because they cannot lose weight rapidly or because they have no results because they eat mountains of food in their eating windows. The ones who do it right are inspirational successes.

Amanda's Fasting Story

I'm not sure where I first heard about IF. Probably some celebrity inspired me. Generally, I hate diets, and I would never have undergone this type of nutritional restriction. I believe in enjoying life and eating when you want to. But I had several health problems, including being overweight. I was actually thirty pounds overweight. Plus, my previous attempts to not eat after 6 o'clock didn't work at all but using IF, I have lost all thirty pounds.

I read that you should go for 10 to 20 hours without eating. So, I chose to go 16 hours without eating as a nice middle ground. Thus, I eat at 5 pm and then go to bed and have breakfast at eight. Obviously, it's worked for me.

But I will tell you what was so hard. The hard part was not eating a nighttime meal. I had to get over that and just sip hot chicory tea. That's a lifesaver, by the way. I love chicory tea. I miss milk, but I use tea and water to fill the 15-16 fasting hours. I keep myself busy and sleep like a baby. It helped me get over the need to snack before bed. Now I enjoy my meals so much more. They are not a routine or chore to fix, but a pleasure that I look forward to.

I loved how adjustable it is, too. One time I had a late office dinner. Easy enough, I just switched breakfast to be at 11 am. It works seamlessly with your schedule. Just keep on top of the hours, and you're good.

During my first month, I dropped ten pounds. Whoohoo! It showed right away. People kept giving me compliments. I didn't mean for these awesome results; they just happened. I didn't have any food restrictions, and I didn't hate my life. I just had to watch when I ate. That's all.

And, my stomach has decreased in inches. I can fit old dresses again! I eat smaller portions as a result. The minute I get full, I don't want to eat anymore. I eat in the morning, but I usually don't want to, I chew to get my calories. I have lost edema in most of my body, and my blood pressure is normal. I sleep better because of the chicory, too. I have no more constipation or stomach pain. I recommend this approach for everyone, and I think everyone should adhere to it as much as possible. It's a great program that works with your body.

Rose`s Fasting Story

By accident, I found out about the 16/8 fasting system, and I researched it thoroughly. I also asked friends and acquaintances. They had all loved it. So, I decided to try it out for myself and share what happened.

So far, I've been doing this plan for three weeks. I have already lost ten pounds. I fast for 16 hours and then eat for eight hours. The fasting starts after I eat dinner and lasts for 16 hours until I have breakfast. Generally, I eat at 8 pm and then again at noon. I just adjust the times if I eat earlier or later. It is so simple; anyone can do it. I don't have tons of eating restrictions, but I do eat more protein now. For the 16 hours, my body just rests and cleanses.

At first, it was pretty difficult. I was taught that breakfast is the most important meal of the day, so I felt like I was committing some sin when I would go to work without breakfast in my belly. My whole life, I would eat a big breakfast of cereal, boiled eggs, sandwiches, and even a smoothie. Giving it up made me feel like something was wrong. For a few days, my schedule was all out-of-whack, and I was incredibly hungry by lunchtime. By the end of a week, though, that all passed. I began to feel lighter and not look at the clock waiting for noon.

You don't have to skip breakfast, by the way. That's just what I did. You can eat in the morning and eat dinner earlier. If you need your morning meal, do it. That's what is great about this system; you can make it work for you. I can honestly say that I don't miss breakfast much, though.

You don't have to give up the foods you love. You can still eat your favorite dessert! I love chocolate, so I eat that during my window. What diet allows you to do that??? Uh, this one! But this plan isn't really a diet, just a power system. I feel light, and I'm losing fat, not muscle mass. Don't torture yourself with fad diets that don't work; use this power system and enjoy the results. IF is really just a simple lifestyle change you can fit into your daily life.

Ellice's Fasting Story

I had pretty much given up on remission from rheumatoid arthritis after giving birth. I was on the verge of despair, both physically and mentally. My quality of life was so low. Drug treatments don't work well for me, and my family has a long history of Type 1 Diabetes. I knew that I would develop diabetes because of the sudden jumps my pancreas was doing. I knew that something was wrong because I would break out in cold sweats and then feel terrible weakness until I ate. I didn't know what to do, and my options seemed nonexistent.

But on some baby board, I found some women raving about IF. Well, why not try it? Nothing else was working.

I started experimenting with it. It wasn't so bad. I have started going longer times with my fasts. Recently, I made it 36 hours! I noticed that after starting this practice, I felt way better in the mornings. Usually, I hurt the worst in my joints at this time, so the pain was subsiding. One day about a week in, I woke up feeling light, like my depression had lifted. Then I realized that I hadn't eaten since 4 pm the day before. I was distracted and forgot supper. I guess that happens, but it showed me that I don't need three meals a day as they say.

A light bulb went off in my head. If I didn't have so much protein in my body from dinner, maybe my body could not spare so much for autoimmune processes. Or maybe if my organs were resting and not moving so much with digestion, so they did not make so many extra movements and enzymes. Maybe my body was getting rid of toxins. Perhaps this approach was the secret to getting well from my RA.

So now I do IF and I restrict my solid food, but I drink all the water I want. Over three months, my condition has improved a lot; I'm a lot more flexible, and I have no more reflux esophagitis!

The only bad thing is that I have to stick with this for life. I broke my regimen once, and my symptoms flared up like clockwork. This plan will be for life. But it's not so bad. It is super easy to follow. The elders knew something when they said not to eat after 6!

Jane's Fasting Story

A bit about me. I hit 210 pounds (I'm 5'6"
and 28 so yeah, I was obese) and I hated looking at
myself in photos or the mirror. I was humiliated by
the scale in the doctor's office. I knew that it was
time to do something.

I tried a bunch of diets — even keto. I
couldn't follow them long enough to see long-term
results. My friend said I was losing mostly water
weight. I decided to try IF at her suggestion, fasting
16/8. So, I eat between 9 and 5 and then I don't eat
from 5 to 9. This schedule works since I go to work
at 10 so I can grab breakfast and feel fulfilled as I
work.

The weight loss has been slow but sure —
definitely a minus for IF but it's still weight loss and
it's healthier than starving yourself. I believe you
should lose no more than 10 pounds per month and
that's what I've been doing. I'm glad I tried this
approach, and I recommend it to anyone.

Melissa`s Fasting Story

IF was perfect for me, since I have problems with breakfast. I chose to eat from 12-8 and not eat from 8-12. I barely notice that I'm fasting since I'm mostly asleep then. I have lost 7 pounds in a month, just sleeping when I don't eat. It's terrifically easy. No diet to follow, either.

The only minus is that sometimes I can't meet my caloric intake. I just don't have time. I am using FatSecret and trying to meet my quota.

Candace's Fasting Story

I was fifty pounds overweight, and then I got the worst news: My cholesterol was high, and my fasting blood sugar was 190. The doctor said I was in pre-diabetes. I was only 32! And I had a little boy at home to worry about. The idea of losing everything to diabetes scared me, so I knew I needed to change. I looked into diets ideal for pre-diabetics, and something about intermittent fasting came up. I looked into it more and decided to start.

No lie, it was not easy. I am used to getting up throughout the night to snack. My favorite hobby is relaxing at home with my husband and eating lots of snacks, too. And we love to go out and eat whenever we're hungry. I had to learn a lot of discipline and control. I started by not eating for 16 hours and didn't think I could do it. I tried eating a teaspoon of almond butter and drinking water when I felt hungry, and that really helped.

Well, now I'm eight pounds from my goal weight, meaning I've lost 42 pounds in the past six months. My cholesterol is better, and my doctor says I am no longer pre-diabetic. Plus, I feel better. I have more energy to play with my little boy and for my husband. Our sex life is so much better. He has lost weight doing this plan with me, too, and we are so happy.

Conclusion

Your first and biggest takeaway from this book is to talk to your doctor before starting this diet. You don't want to do anything that jeopardizes your health!

The second is to be careful about what sources you follow as you begin this journey. There are tons of sources, not all of them good. Be sure to look into the scientific research and the credentials of the author behind a source.

Your life will alter dramatically with intermittent fasting. You can stave off cancer and dementia. You can halt aging. You can lose weight. You can reverse Type 2 Diabetes, or at least manage it more successfully. Years of crash dieting and starving yourself will not get you the results that intermittent fasting can, in a shorter time.

Start slow. Find the plan that works for you and work up to it. Listen to your body. Have a support group, but keep it to yourself. Use a journal.

Also, make your eating windows count with healthy food. Several healthy options and recipes can make your eating windows, both enjoyable and nourishing. This approach is not about starving yourself, but instead feeding yourself and then letting your body cleanse. Intermittent fasting calls for working with your body's natural cycles and processes for great results.

IF is not a diet, but rather a way of eating, you can keep it up for your entire life. It offers a sustainable approach to continue to keep the weight off, and the health benefits up. Basically, it is just a routine that works with your body. You can expect to see results of up to two pounds in a week, depending on the amount of weight you carry. However, even when you have hit your goal weight, you must continue following the plan. Otherwise, you will return to your former weight and lose all of the health benefits that you have gained. Consider IF like a new habit that helps you gain health, not a fad diet that makes you lose weight.

Look back and feel proud of yourself. Realize how much better you feel and look. Peruse old photos and compare them to what you see in the mirror today. Revel in the compliments you get: "You've lost weight!" "Your skin is glowing!" "You seem so much happier now." The ease of this way of eating can really make you want to stick with it.

Notes

1. *Denial is the New Indulgence for Elites*. Quartz. https://qz.com/1098242/silicon-valleys-fasting-craze-is-proof-that-self-denial-is-the-new-indulgence-for-elites/.

Levine, Beth & Klionsky, Daniel. (2017). Autophagy wins the 2016 Nobel Prize in Physiology or Medicine: Breakthroughs in baker's yeast fuel advances in biomedical research Proc Natl Acad Sci U S A. 2017 Jan 10; 114(2): 201–205. Published online 2016 Dec 30. doi: 10.1073/pnas.1619876114

2. Martin, Bowen, et al. *Caloric restriction and intermittent fasting: Two potential diets for successful brain aging*. Ageing Res Rev. Published in final edited form as Ageing Res Rev. 2006 Aug; 5(3): 332–353. Published online 2006 Aug 8. doi: 10.1016/j.arr.2006.04.002.

3. Diet Review: Intermittent Fasting for Weight Loss. *Harvard School of Public Health*. https://www.hsph.harvard.edu/nutritionsource/healthy-weight/diet-reviews/intermittent-fasting/.

4. Fung, Jason, Dr. *How to Renew Your Body: Fasting and Autophagy*. Diet Doctor. https://www.dietdoctor.com/renew-body-fasting-autophagy.

5. Oh, T., et al. *Body Weight Fluctuations and Incident Diabetes Mellitus, Cardiovascular Disease, and Mortality: A 16-Year Prospective Cohort*

Study. Journal of Clinical Endocrinology and Metabolism, Volume 104, Issue 3, March 2019, Pages 639–646, https://doi.org/10.1210/jc.2018-01239.

6. Wayne, Minnie. *The Benefits of Intermittent Fasting for Your Well-Being and for Strength. https://physicaliq.com/intermittent-fasting-for-your-wellbeing-and-for-strength/*

7. Johnson JB[1], Summer W, Cutler RG, Martin B, Hyun DH, Dixit VD, Pearson M, Nassar M, Telljohann R, Maudsley S, Carlson O, John S, Laub DR, Mattson MP. *Alternate day calorie restriction improves clinical findings and reduces markers of oxidative stress and inflammation in overweight adults with moderate asthma.* Free Radic Biol Med. 2007 Mar 1;42(5):665-74. Epub 2006 Dec 14.

8. Anu Rahal, et al. *Oxidative Stress, Prooxidants, and Antioxidants: The Interplay. BioMed Research International,* Volume 2014, Article ID 761264, 19 pages, http://dx.doi.org/10.1155/2014/761264.

9. Antoni, R., et al. *The Effects of Intermittent Energy Restriction on Indices of Cardiometabolic Health.* Research in Endocrinology, Volume 2014 (2014), Article ID 459119, 24 pages, DOI: 10.5171/2014.459119.

10. Dr. Maggie Ney. *Intermittent Fasting and Your Hormones.* Alaska Center for Integrative Medicine. https://akashacenter.com/intermittent-fasting-and-your-hormones/

11. Jason, Amanda. *Intermittent Fasting for Women: The Essential Beginners Guide for Weight Loss, Burn Fat, Heal Your Body Through The Self-Cleansing Process of Autophagy and Live a Healthy Lifestyle*. Amazon Publishing. ASIN: B07K2JG6DV.

12. Michos, Erin, MD. *Why Cholesterol Matters for Women*. Health. https://www.hopkinsmedicine.org/health/wellness-and-prevention/why-cholesterol-matters-for-women.

13. Whittel, Naomi. *Glow15: A Science-Based Plan to Lose Weight, Revitalize Your Skin, and Invigorate Your Life*. Houghton Mifflin Harcourt. ISBN-13: 978-1328897671.

14. Gillapsy, Becky. *Losing Weight After 50: Strategies and Food Swaps that Work*. Dr. Becky. https://www.drbeckyfitness.com/category/menopause-weight-loss/

15. Ahmed, A.M. *History of Diabetes Mellitus*. Saudi Medical Journal, 2002, 23 (4), pp. 373-8. DOI: https://www.ncbi.nlm.nih.gov/pubmed/11953758.

16. Karamanou, Mariana, Koutsilieris, Michael, Laios, Konstantinos, et al. *Apollinaire Bouchardat (1806-1886): founder of modern Diabetology*. HORMONES, 2014, 13(2):296-300.

Made in United States
North Haven, CT
28 May 2022

19620920R00059